Dash Diet Cookbook for beginners

Recover the secret of lowering your blood pressure naturally

Favor Leroux

Table of contents

Introduction to the Dash Diet

Sarah was passionate about health and nutrition. As a certified dietitian, she dedicated her life to helping people make better food choices and lead healthier lifestyles. One day, while browsing through the cookbook section of her local bookstore, she came across a popular Dash Diet Cookbook for beginners.

The Dash Diet, known for its emphasis on fruits, vegetables, lean proteins, and whole grains, was a favorite among those looking to improve their heart health and manage their weight. However, as Sarah flipped through the pages of the cookbook, she couldn't help but notice some inaccuracies and inconsistencies in the recipes and meal plans.

Determined to make a difference, Sarah decided to revise the Dash Diet Cookbook herself. Armed with her knowledge and expertise, she meticulously went through each recipe, ensuring that they were not only delicious but also nutritious and aligned with the principles of the Dash Diet.

She replaced processed ingredients with whole foods, reduced the amount of added sugars and salt, and increased the variety of fruits and vegetables in the recipes. Sarah also included helpful tips and guidelines for beginners, making it easier for them to understand and follow the Dash Diet successfully.

After weeks of hard work, Sarah finally completed the revised edition of the Dash Diet Cookbook for beginners. Excited to share her creation with the world, she reached out to publishers and soon found one who was eager to release her book.

The revised cookbook quickly gained popularity, receiving rave reviews from both beginners and seasoned Dash Dieters alike. People praised Sarah for her dedication to accuracy and her ability to make healthy eating accessible and enjoyable for everyone.

As the sales of the cookbook soared, Sarah's impact on the health and well-being of others grew exponentially. She continued to inspire people to embrace the Dash Diet and adopt healthier eating habits, one delicious recipe at a time. And through her passion and expertise, Sarah proved that with the right diet, anyone can achieve their health goals and live their best life.

1.1 Origins of the Dash Diet

The origins of the Dash diet can be traced back to a research study conducted in the early 1990s called the Dietary Approaches to Stop Hypertension (DASH) trial. This groundbreaking study aimed to investigate the effects of different dietary patterns on blood pressure, specifically focusing on individuals with hypertension.

The DASH trial was sponsored by the National Heart, Lung, and Blood Institute (NHLBI) and involved over 450 participants. The participants were divided into three groups: one group followed a typical American diet, another group followed a diet rich in fruits and vegetables, and the third group followed a diet that combined elements of both diets.

The results of the study were remarkable. It was found that the group following the diet rich in fruits and vegetables experienced significant reductions in blood pressure compared to those following the typical American diet. This led to further research and development of what is now known as the Dash diet.

Since its inception, the Dash diet has gained recognition as an effective approach for reducing high blood pressure and promoting overall health. It has been endorsed by various health organizations, including the

NHLBI, American Heart Association (AHA), and World Health Organization (WHO).

1.2 Key Principles of the Dash Diet

The key principles of the Dash diet revolve around consuming nutrient-rich foods while limiting sodium intake. The diet emphasizes a balanced eating plan that includes:

1.Fruits and Vegetables: The Dash diet encourages individuals to consume a variety of fruits and vegetables daily. These foods are rich in essential vitamins, minerals, antioxidants, and fiber, which contribute to overall health and well-being.

2.Whole Grains: Whole grains such as brown rice, whole wheat bread, oats, quinoa, and barley are an important part of the Dash diet. They provide complex carbohydrates for sustained energy levels and are a good source of fiber, which aids in digestion and helps maintain a healthy weight.

3.Lean Proteins: The Dash diet promotes the consumption of lean proteins such as skinless poultry, fish, beans, lentils, and tofu. These protein sources are low in saturated fat and provide essential amino acids for muscle growth and repair.

4.Low-Fat Dairy Products: The Dash diet encourages the consumption of low-fat dairy products like skim milk, yogurt, and cheese. These foods are rich in calcium and vitamin D, which are important for bone health.

5.Limited Sodium Intake: One of the key principles of the Dash diet is to limit sodium intake to no more than

2,300 milligrams per day (or 1,500 milligrams for individuals with hypertension or at risk for it). This involves reducing the consumption of processed foods, canned soups, fast food, and adding less salt during cooking or at the table.

By following these key principles, individuals can lower their blood pressure levels and reduce the risk of heart disease. The Dash diet provides a flexible framework that can be adapted to individual preferences and dietary needs.

1.3 Scientific Evidence Supporting the Effectiveness of the Dash Diet

Numerous scientific studies have provided strong evidence supporting the effectiveness of the Dash diet in reducing high blood pressure and improving overall health outcomes.

A study published in The New England Journal of Medicine compared four different diets: a typical American diet; a typical American diet supplemented with fruits and vegetables; a Dash-like diet with added fruits and vegetables; and a Dash-like diet without added fruits and vegetables. The results showed that both versions of the Dash-like diets significantly lowered blood pressure compared to the typical American diet.

Another study published in Circulation found that adherence to the Dash diet was associated with a reduced risk of developing heart failure among middle-aged women. The study followed over 36,000 women for an average of 10 years and found that those who closely followed the Dash diet had a 37% lower risk of heart failure compared to those who did not.

Furthermore, a meta-analysis published in the American Journal of Hypertension analyzed data from 15 studies and concluded that the Dash diet significantly reduced both systolic and diastolic blood pressure. The analysis also found that the Dash diet was effective in lowering blood pressure regardless of age, sex, or race.

These are just a few examples of the scientific evidence supporting the effectiveness of the Dash diet. The consistent findings across multiple studies highlight its potential to improve cardiovascular health and overall well-being.

In conclusion, the origins of the Dash diet can be traced back to the DASH trial conducted in the early 1990s. The key principles of the Dash diet revolve around consuming nutrient-rich foods while limiting sodium intake. Scientific evidence has consistently shown that following the Dash diet can lead to significant reductions in blood pressure and a decreased risk of heart disease. By incorporating these principles into your daily life, you can take control of your health and make positive changes that will last a lifetime.

Chapter 2:

Understanding the Dash Diet

2.1 Incorporating nutrient-rich foods into your daily meals

Incorporating nutrient-rich foods into your daily meals is essential for maintaining good health and well-being. Here are some tips for doing so:

Prioritize whole foods: Choose whole, minimally processed foods over highly processed ones. Whole foods such as fruits, vegetables, whole grains, lean proteins, nuts, and seeds are packed with essential nutrients like vitamins, minerals, fiber, and antioxidants.

Include a variety of colorful fruits and vegetables: Different colors in fruits and vegetables signify different nutrients, so aim to include a variety of colors in your meals. For example, leafy greens like spinach and kale are rich in vitamin K and folate, while orange and yellow fruits and vegetables like carrots and oranges provide beta-carotene and vitamin C.

Opt for lean proteins: Incorporate lean protein sources such as poultry, fish, tofu, legumes, and beans into your meals. These foods are not only rich in protein but also provide important nutrients like iron, zinc, and B vitamins.

Choose whole grains: Replace refined grains with whole grains like brown rice, quinoa, oats, and whole wheat bread. Whole grains contain more fiber, vitamins, and minerals compared to refined grains, which have been stripped of many nutrients during processing.

Add healthy fats to your diet: Add foods like avocados, almonds, seeds, and olive oil—which are good sources of fat—to your meals.These fats provide essential fatty acids that are important for brain health, hormone production, and absorption of fat-soluble vitamins.

Don't forget about dairy or dairy alternatives: Dairy products like milk, yogurt, and cheese are good sources of calcium, protein, and other nutrients. If you're lactose intolerant or prefer plant-based options, choose fortified dairy alternatives like almond milk or soy yogurt.

Snack on nutrient-rich foods: Instead of reaching for processed snacks, choose nutrient-rich options like fresh fruit, raw vegetables with hummus, Greek yogurt, or a handful of nuts and seeds.

Stay hydrated: Remember to drink plenty of water throughout the day, as hydration is crucial for overall health and well-being. You can also incorporate hydrating foods like cucumbers, watermelon, and celery into your meals and snacks.

By incorporating these nutrient-rich foods into your daily meals, you can ensure that you're getting the essential nutrients your body needs to thrive. Additionally, focusing on variety and balance will help you maintain a healthy and enjoyable eating pattern.

2.2 Reducing sodium intake in your diet

Reducing sodium intake is important for maintaining good health, as excessive sodium consumption is linked to high blood pressure, heart disease, and other health issues. Here are some tips for reducing sodium intake in your diet:

Read food labels: Pay attention to the sodium content listed on food labels when grocery shopping. Whenever feasible, choose products with labels that say "low sodium," "reduced sodium," or "no added salt".

Cook at home: Cooking meals at home allows you to control the amount of salt added to your food. Use herbs, spices, citrus juices, and vinegar to enhance flavor without relying on salt.

Limit processed foods: Processed and packaged foods such as canned soups, frozen meals, deli meats, and snack foods often contain high amounts of sodium. Opt for fresh, whole foods instead.

Choose fresh or frozen vegetables: Fresh or frozen vegetables are naturally low in sodium compared to canned varieties, which are often packed in salted water or brine. If you do choose canned vegetables, look for options labeled as "low sodium" or "no salt added."

Use salt substitutes cautiously: While salt substitutes can be lower in sodium or even sodium-free, they may contain other ingredients like potassium chloride, which can be harmful to individuals with certain medical conditions. Consult with a healthcare provider before using salt substitutes.

Rinse canned foods: If you use canned beans, vegetables, or other canned foods, rinse them under running water before consuming to reduce their sodium content.

Be mindful of condiments and sauces: Condiments like soy sauce, ketchup, barbecue sauce, and salad dressings can be high in sodium. Choose low-sodium or reduced-sodium versions, or make your own using fresh ingredients.

Limit eating out: Restaurant meals and fast food tend to be high in sodium due to added salt and other flavor enhancers. When dining out, ask for dishes to be prepared without added salt or request sauces and dressings on the side so you can control how much you use.

Gradually reduce salt: Gradually reduce the amount of salt you add to your meals to allow your taste buds to adjust to lower sodium levels over time.

By following these tips and being mindful of your sodium intake, you can reduce your risk of health problems associated with high sodium consumption and promote overall well-being.

Chapter 3:

The Benefits of the Dash Diet

3.1 Lowering high blood pressure

Lowering high blood pressure (hypertension) is crucial for reducing the risk of heart disease, stroke, and other health complications. Here are some effective strategies for managing and

lowering high blood pressure:Healthy Diet: Follow a balanced diet rich in fruits, vegetables, whole grains, lean proteins, and low-fat dairy products. This dietary pattern, known as the DASH (Dietary Approaches to Stop Hypertension) diet, emphasizes foods high in potassium, magnesium, and calcium while limiting sodium intake.

Reduce Sodium Intake: Limit the amount of sodium in your diet by avoiding processed foods, canned soups, fast food, and salty snacks. Opt for fresh, whole foods and use herbs, spices, and other flavorings to season your meals instead of salt.

Maintain a Healthy Weight: Aim for a healthy weight by incorporating regular physical activity into your routine and making dietary changes to support weight loss if needed. Losing even a small amount of weight can help lower blood pressure.

Regular Exercise: Engage in regular aerobic exercise such as brisk walking, jogging, cycling, or swimming for at least 150 minutes per week, or about 30 minutes most days of the week. Additionally, incorporate strength training exercises at least two days per week.

Limit Alcohol: Limit alcohol consumption to moderate levels, which means up to one drink per day for women and up to two drinks per day for men. Excessive alcohol intake can raise blood pressure and contribute to other health problems.

Quit Smoking: If you smoke, quit smoking as soon as possible. Smoking damages blood vessels and increases the risk of heart disease and stroke. Quitting smoking can significantly lower blood pressure and improve overall health.

Manage Stress: Practice stress-reducing techniques such as deep breathing, meditation, yoga, tai chi, or spending time on hobbies and activities you enjoy. Chronic stress can contribute to high blood pressure, so finding healthy ways to manage stress is important.

Monitor Blood Pressure Regularly: Keep track of your blood pressure at home using a home blood pressure monitor. Regular monitoring can help you and your healthcare provider assess the effectiveness of your treatment plan and make necessary adjustments.

Medication: In some cases, medication may be necessary to lower blood pressure, especially if lifestyle changes alone are not sufficient. Work with your healthcare provider to determine the most appropriate medication regimen for your individual needs.
By incorporating these lifestyle changes and working closely with your healthcare provider, you can effectively manage and lower high blood pressure, reducing your risk of serious health complications.

3.2 Reducing the risk of heart disease

Reducing the risk of heart disease involves adopting a heart-healthy lifestyle and making choices that support cardiovascular health. Here are some key strategies for reducing the risk of heart disease:

Eat a Heart-Healthy Diet: Focus on a diet rich in fruits, vegetables, whole grains, lean proteins (such as fish, poultry, beans, and legumes), and healthy fats (such as those found in avocados, nuts, seeds, and olive oil). Limit saturated fats, trans fats, cholesterol, sodium, and added sugars.

Maintain a Healthy Weight: Aim for a body mass index (BMI) within the healthy range (18.5 to 24.9). Achieving and maintaining a healthy weight reduces the risk of high blood pressure, high cholesterol, and type 2 diabetes, all of which are risk factors for heart disease.

Engage in Regular Physical Activity: Aim for at least 150 minutes of moderate-intensity aerobic exercise or 75 minutes of vigorous-intensity aerobic exercise per week, along with muscle-strengthening activities on two or more days per week. Regular exercise helps maintain a healthy weight, lowers blood pressure and cholesterol, and improves overall cardiovascular health.

Quit Smoking and Avoid Secondhand Smoke: Smoking is a major risk factor for heart disease. If you smoke, quit smoking as soon as possible, and avoid exposure to secondhand smoke.

Limit Alcohol Intake: Limit alcohol consumption to moderate levels, which means up to one drink per day for women and up to two drinks per day for men. Excessive alcohol consumption can raise blood pressure, increase triglyceride levels, and contribute to obesity, all of which are risk factors for heart disease.

Manage Stress: Chronic stress can contribute to heart disease risk. Practice stress-reducing techniques such as deep breathing, meditation, yoga, tai chi, or engaging in hobbies and activities you enjoy.

Get Quality Sleep: Aim for 7-9 hours of quality sleep per night. Poor sleep quality or insufficient sleep is associated with an increased risk of heart disease and other health problems.

Monitor Blood Pressure and Cholesterol Levels: Regularly monitor your blood pressure and cholesterol levels, and work with your healthcare provider to manage them within healthy ranges. High blood pressure and high cholesterol are major risk factors for heart disease.

Manage Chronic Conditions: If you have diabetes, high blood pressure, high cholesterol, or other chronic conditions, work with your healthcare provider to manage them effectively through medication, lifestyle changes, and regular monitoring.

Regular Health Check-Ups: Schedule regular check-ups with your healthcare provider to assess your overall health, screen for risk factors, and discuss preventive measures.
By incorporating these strategies into your daily life, you can significantly reduce your risk of heart disease and promote long-term cardiovascular health.

Chapter 4:

Healthy and Flavorful Dinner Options

4.1 Grilled salmon with roasted vegetables

Grilled salmon with roasted vegetables is a delicious and nutritious dish that's easy to prepare. Here's a simple recipe:

Ingredients:

4 salmon filets

2 bell peppers (any color), sliced

1 zucchini, sliced

1 yellow squash, sliced

1 red onion, sliced

2 tablespoons olive oil

Salt and pepper to taste

2 cloves garlic, minced

1 teaspoon dried thyme

1 teaspoon dried rosemary

Lemon wedges for serving

Instructions:

Preheat your grill to medium-high heat.

In a large bowl, toss the sliced bell peppers, zucchini, yellow squash, and red onion with olive oil, minced garlic, dried thyme, dried rosemary, salt, and pepper until evenly coated.

Arrange the vegetables in a single layer on a baking sheet..

Place the baking sheet on the grill and roast the vegetables, turning occasionally, until they are tender and slightly charred, about 15-20 minutes.
While the vegetables are roasting, season the salmon filets with salt and pepper.

Place the salmon filets directly on the grill and cook for about 4-5 minutes per side, or until the salmon is cooked through and flakes easily with a fork.
Once the salmon and vegetables are done, remove them from the grill.

Serve the grilled salmon with the roasted vegetables alongside lemon wedges for squeezing over the top.
Enjoy your delicious and healthy meal!
Feel free to adjust the seasoning or vegetables according to your taste preferences. This dish pairs well with rice, quinoa, or a fresh green salad.

4.2 Quinoa-stuffed bell peppers

Quinoa-stuffed bell peppers are a nutritious and flavorful vegetarian dish. Here's a recipe to make them:

Ingredients:
4 large bell peppers (any color), halved and seeds removed
1 cup quinoa, rinsed

2 cups vegetable broth or water
1 tablespoon olive oil
1 onion, diced
2 cloves garlic, minced
1 zucchini, diced
1 cup diced tomatoes (fresh or canned)
1 cup cooked black beans (or canned, drained and rinsed)
1 teaspoon ground cumin
1 teaspoon smoked paprika
Salt and pepper to taste
1 cup shredded cheese (optional)
Chopped fresh cilantro or parsley for garnish

Instructions:

Preheat your oven to 375°F (190°C).

In a medium saucepan, bring the vegetable broth (or water) to a boil. Add the quinoa, reduce heat to low, cover, and simmer for about 15 minutes, or until the quinoa is cooked and fluffy. Remove from heat and set aside.

Heat the olive oil in a big skillet over medium heat while the quinoa cooks. Add the chopped onion and simmer for about 5 minutes, or until transparent. Cook the minced garlic for one to two more minutes after adding it.

Add diced zucchini to the skillet and cook for 3-4 minutes, until slightly softened.

Stir in diced tomatoes, cooked black beans, ground cumin, smoked paprika, salt, and pepper. Allow the

flavors to combine by cooking for a further two to three minutes.
In a large mixing bowl, combine the cooked quinoa with the vegetable mixture until well combined.

Place the bell pepper halves in a baking dish, cut side up. Fill each bell pepper half with the quinoa and vegetable mixture, pressing down gently to pack it in.
Top each stuffed pepper with shredded cheese, if you'd like.
Bake the baking dish in the preheated oven for 25 to 30 minutes, or until the peppers are soft, covered with aluminum foil.
Remove the foil and bake for an additional 5 minutes, or until the cheese is melted and bubbly.

Before serving, garnish with freshly cut parsley or cilantro.

Enjoy your delicious quinoa-stuffed bell peppers as a healthy and satisfying meal!
Feel free to customize the stuffing with your favorite vegetables or spices to suit your taste preferences. These stuffed peppers also make great leftovers for lunch the next day!

4.3 Lemon garlic chicken with asparagus

Lemon garlic chicken with asparagus is a flavorful and wholesome dish. Here's a recipe to make it:

Ingredients:
4 boneless, skinless chicken breasts
Salt and pepper to taste
2 tablespoons olive oil
4 cloves garlic, minced
1 teaspoon dried oregano
1 teaspoon dried thyme
Zest and juice of 1 lemon
1 bunch asparagus, trimmed
Lemon slices for garnish
Chopped fresh parsley for garnish
Instructions:
Preheat your oven to 400°F (200°C).
Sprinkle salt and pepper on both sides of the chicken breasts.
Heat the olive oil in a sizable oven-safe skillet over medium-high heat.

.Add the seasoned chicken breasts to the skillet and cook for 3-4 minutes on each side, or until golden brown.
Remove the chicken breasts from the skillet and set aside on a plate.
Add the minced garlic to the same skillet and cook it for about one minute, or until fragrant..
Add dried oregano, dried thyme, lemon zest, and lemon juice to the skillet. Stir to combine, scraping up any browned bits from the bottom of the skillet.

Add the trimmed asparagus to the skillet and toss to coat with the lemon garlic mixture.

Return the chicken breasts to the skillet, nestling them among the asparagus.

After transferring the skillet to the oven, warm it and bake for 15 to 20 minutes, or until the asparagus is soft and the chicken is cooked through.

After that, take the skillet out of the oven. Add lemon slices and finely chopped fresh parsley as garnish.
Serve the lemon garlic chicken with asparagus hot, alongside your favorite side dishes such as rice, quinoa, or mashed potatoes.

Enjoy your delicious and flavorful meal!
Feel free to adjust the seasoning or add other herbs and spices to suit your taste preferences. This dish is easy to customize and makes for a satisfying dinner option.

Chapter 5:

Snacks and Appetizers for Any Occasion

5.1 Hummus and veggie platter

A hummus and veggie platter is a classic and healthy appetizer or snack option. Here's how you can put together a delicious platter:

***Ingredients*:**
1 cup hummus (store-bought or homemade)
Assorted fresh vegetables, such as:
Carrot sticks
Cucumber slices
Bell pepper strips (any color)
Cherry tomatoes
Celery sticks
Snap peas
Radishes
Optional extras:
Olives
Pickles
Roasted chickpeas
Pita bread or pita chips
Sliced bread or crackers
Lemon wedges

Fresh herbs for garnish, such as parsley or cilantro
Olive oil extra virgin to drizzle
Salt and pepper to taste
Instructions:
Prepare the fresh vegetables by washing and cutting them into sticks, slices, or bite-sized pieces. Arrange them on a large serving platter or tray.
Place the hummus in a bowl and place it in the center of the platter.
If using any optional extras like olives or pickles, arrange them around the hummus bowl or scatter them throughout the platter.
If serving with pita bread or pita chips, arrange them on the platter or serve them in a separate bowl.

Sprinkle some salt and pepper over the vegetables, if desired, or provide salt and pepper shakers for guests to season to their liking.

Garnish the platter with fresh herbs, such as parsley or cilantro, for a pop of color and added flavor.
Drizzle a little extra virgin olive oil over the hummus, if desired, for extra richness.
Serve the hummus and veggie platter immediately, accompanied by lemon wedges for squeezing over the vegetables if desired.
Enjoy your delicious and nutritious snack or appetizer!

This platter is not only visually appealing but also provides a variety of textures and flavors to enjoy. It's perfect for parties, gatherings, or as a light and healthy snack any time of the day.

5.2 Caprese skewers with balsamic glaze

Caprese skewers with balsamic glaze are a delightful appetizer or party snack that combines the classic flavors of fresh mozzarella, ripe tomatoes, basil, and balsamic vinegar. Here's how to make them:

Ingredients:
Fresh mozzarella balls (bocconcini), drained
Cherry tomatoes
Fresh basil leaves
Balsamic glaze (store-bought or homemade)
Bamboo skewers or toothpicks
Instructions:
Begin by preparing the ingredients. Drain the fresh mozzarella balls if they are stored in liquid. Wash and dry the cherry tomatoes and fresh basil leaves.

To assemble the skewers, thread one cherry tomato onto a skewer, followed by a fresh basil leaf folded in half, and then a mozzarella ball. Repeat this pattern until the skewer is filled, leaving a little space at the end for easy handling.

Arrange the assembled Caprese skewers on a serving platter or tray.
After assembling all of the skewers, brush them with balsamic glaze.You can either use store-bought

balsamic glaze or make your own by reducing balsamic vinegar in a saucepan until it thickens into a syrupy consistency.If desired, you can sprinkle a pinch of salt and freshly ground black pepper over the skewers for extra flavor.

Serve the Caprese skewers immediately, garnished with additional fresh basil leaves if desired.

Enjoy these delicious and elegant appetizers as a light and refreshing addition to any gathering or party!

Caprese skewers with balsamic glaze are not only visually appealing but also bursting with flavor. They make a perfect finger food option for cocktail parties, potlucks, or any occasion where you want to impress your guests with minimal effort.

5.3 Sweet potato fries with spicy yogurt dip

Sweet potato fries with spicy yogurt dip make for a tasty and healthier alternative to traditional fries. Here's how to make them:

Ingredients for Sweet Potato Fries:

Peel and chop two big sweet potatoes into fries.

Two tsp olive oil

1 teaspoon paprika

1/2 teaspoon garlic powder

Salt and pepper to taste

Ingredients for Spicy Yogurt Dip:

1 cup Greek yogurt

1 tablespoon Sriracha sauce (adjust to taste for desired level of spiciness)

1 tablespoon honey

1 tablespoon lime juice

Salt and pepper to taste

Instructions:Preheat your oven to 425°F (220°C) and line a baking sheet with parchment paper.

In a large bowl, toss the sweet potato fries with olive oil, paprika, garlic powder, salt, and pepper until evenly coated.

Spread the sweet potato fries out in a single layer on the prepared baking sheet, making sure they're not overcrowded. This enables them to bake up pleasantly crisp.

Bake the sweet potato fries in the preheated oven for 20-25 minutes, flipping them halfway through, until they are golden brown and crispy.

While the sweet potato fries are baking, prepare the spicy yogurt dip. In a small bowl, whisk together Greek yogurt, Sriracha sauce, honey, lime juice, salt, and pepper until smooth and well combined. Taste and adjust the seasoning or spiciness level according to your preference.Once the sweet potato fries are done baking, remove them from the oven and let them cool slightly.

Serve the sweet potato fries hot, alongside the spicy yogurt dip for dipping.

Enjoy your delicious and flavorful sweet potato fries with spicy yogurt dip as a satisfying snack or side dish!

These sweet potato fries are crispy on the outside, tender on the inside, and perfectly seasoned with a hint of spice. The creamy and tangy yogurt dip adds a delightful contrast and extra flavor.It's an excellent blend that will definitely delight your palate!

Chapter 6:

Mindful Eating and Portion Control

6.1 Understanding the importance of mindful eating
Understanding the importance of mindful eating can lead to numerous benefits for both physical and mental well-being. Mindful eating is a practice that involves paying full attention to the experience of eating and drinking, including the sensations of taste, smell, texture, and the act of chewing and swallowing. Here are several key reasons why mindful eating is important:

Promotes Healthy Eating Habits: Mindful eating encourages individuals to be more aware of their food choices, portion sizes, and hunger cues. By paying attention to the body's signals of hunger and fullness, people are more likely to make healthier food choices and avoid overeating.

Enhances Digestion: Mindful eating involves chewing food thoroughly and savoring each bite. This aids in better digestion by breaking down food more effectively and allowing the body to absorb nutrients more efficiently.

Reduces Overeating and Binge Eating: By tuning into hunger and satiety cues, mindful eating helps prevent overeating and binge eating episodes. It encourages individuals to eat until they are satisfied, rather than eating beyond their body's needs.

Increases Enjoyment of Food: Mindful eating emphasizes the sensory experience of eating, allowing individuals to fully appreciate the flavors, textures, and aromas of their food. Meals may become more satisfying and enjoyable as a result.

Supports Weight Management: Studies have shown that practicing mindful eating can be effective in weight management and weight loss efforts. By fostering a deeper awareness of food intake and eating behaviors, individuals are better equipped to make conscious choices that support their weight goals.

Improves Body Awareness: Mindful eating promotes a greater connection between the mind and body, helping individuals recognize physical hunger and distinguish it from other types of hunger, such as emotional or environmental cues.

Reduces Stress and Anxiety: Mindful eating techniques, such as deep breathing and focusing on the present moment, can help reduce stress and anxiety related to food and eating. It encourages a more relaxed and mindful approach to mealtimes.

Cultivates Gratitude: Mindful eating encourages gratitude for the nourishment and sustenance provided by food. Taking time to acknowledge and appreciate the food on one's plate can foster a deeper sense of gratitude and connection to the food we consume.

Overall, practicing mindful eating can lead to a more balanced and harmonious relationship with food, as well as improved overall health and well-being. By bringing mindfulness to the table, individuals can savor the pleasures of eating while also nourishing their bodies and minds.

6.2 Tips for practicing portion control at meals

Practicing portion control at meals is an effective way to manage weight, improve digestion, and maintain overall health. The following advice will assist you in managing your portions:

Use Smaller Plates: Opt for smaller plates and bowls to help control portion sizes. Research shows that people tend to eat less when they use smaller dishware because it creates the illusion of a larger portion.

Measure and Weigh Food: When portioning out foods like grains, proteins, and fats, use measuring cups, spoons, or a food scale. This can make you more conscious of the right portion sizes and help you avoid overindulging.

Divide Your Plate: Visualize your plate divided into sections: half for vegetables, one-quarter for protein, and one-quarter for grains or starchy foods. This helps ensure a balanced meal with appropriate portions of each food group.

Practice the Hand Method: Use your hand as a guide for portion sizes. For example:

Protein: The size of a serving corresponds to your palm.

Vegetables: Fill half your plate with non-starchy vegetables, aiming for about two handfuls.

Grains: A serving size is about the size of your fist.

Fats: Limit added fats to about the size of your thumb.

Slow Down and Chew Thoroughly: Eating slowly and chewing your food thoroughly gives your body time to recognize when it's full, preventing overeating. Put your utensils down between bites and take time to savor the flavors of your food.

Be Mindful of Liquid Calories: Pay attention to portion sizes of beverages, as liquid calories can add up quickly. Opt for water, herbal tea, or other low-calorie beverages, and be mindful of portion sizes for higher-calorie drinks like juice, soda, and alcohol.

Pre-Portion Snacks: Instead of eating directly from a large bag or container, pre-portion snacks into smaller containers or bags. This helps prevent mindless snacking and allows you to control portion sizes.

Listen to Your Hunger Cues: Pay attention to your body's hunger and fullness cues.Rather to eating until you're really full, eat when you're hungry and quit when you're content.

Practice Conscious Eating: Be present and mindful during meals, focusing on the sensory experience of eating. Avoid distractions like TV, phones, or computers, which can lead to mindless eating and overeating.

Plan Ahead: Plan your meals and snacks in advance, and portion out appropriate serving sizes ahead of time. This can help prevent impulsive eating and ensure you're consuming balanced meals throughout the day.

By incorporating these tips into your daily routine, you can develop healthier eating habits and maintain better control over your portion sizes, leading to improved overall health and well-being.

6.3 Strategies for avoiding overeating and emotional eating

Avoiding overeating and emotional eating involves developing mindful eating habits and implementing strategies to address underlying triggers and emotions. Here are some strategies to help:

Identify Triggers: Pay attention to the situations, emotions, or environmental cues that trigger overeating or emotional eating. Common triggers may include stress, boredom, loneliness, social situations, or certain foods.

Practice Mindful Eating: Be present and attentive while eating, focusing on the sensory experience of food.

Chew slowly, savoring the flavors and textures, and pay attention to hunger and fullness cues. Mindful eating can help prevent overeating by increasing awareness of portion sizes and promoting satisfaction with smaller amounts of food.

Address Emotional Needs: Instead of turning to food for comfort or distraction, find alternative ways to cope with emotions. Engage in activities that help you relax, such as deep breathing, meditation, yoga, journaling, or talking to a friend or therapist. Practice self-care and prioritize activities that nourish your well-being.
Distract Yourself: When the urge to overeat or emotionally eat strikes, distract yourself with a non-food-related activity. Go for a walk, listen to music, take a bath, read a book, or engage in a hobby you enjoy. By shifting your focus away from food, you can reduce the intensity of emotional cravings.

Keep Healthy Snacks Available: Stock your home and workplace with nutritious snacks that you enjoy. Having healthy options readily available makes it easier to make positive food choices when hunger strikes. Choose snacks that are high in fiber, protein, and healthy fats to help keep you satisfied between meals.
Practice Stress Management: Find healthy ways to manage stress and reduce its impact on your eating habits. Incorporate stress-relief techniques into your daily routine, such as exercise, relaxation exercises, time in nature, or spending time with loved ones. Better

general health and the avoidance of emotional eating are two benefits of stress management.

Plan Balanced Meals: Aim to eat balanced meals that include a variety of nutrients, including protein, fiber, healthy fats, and carbohydrates. Eating balanced meals helps stabilize blood sugar levels and reduce cravings for unhealthy foods.
Reduce Food Triggers: If particular foods make you prone to overindulging or emotional eating, you might want to cut back on how often you eat them.. Keep trigger foods out of the house or practice portion control when consuming them in social situations.

Seek Support: Reach out to friends, family members, or a therapist for support if you're struggling with overeating or emotional eating. Talking to someone you trust can provide encouragement, guidance, and accountability as you work towards healthier eating habits.
Practice Self-Compassion: Be kind to yourself and practice self-compassion when faced with challenges or setbacks. Remember that nobody is perfect, and it's okay to have occasional slip-ups. Focus on progress rather than perfection, and celebrate your successes along the way.By incorporating these strategies into your daily life, you can develop healthier eating habits, reduce overeating and emotional eating, and cultivate a more balanced relationship with food and your emotions.

Conclusion

In conclusion, the Dash Diet Cookbook for beginners not only serves as a gateway to healthier eating but also represents a pivotal moment in the quest for optimal well-being. With its emphasis on the right diet, this cookbook becomes a transformative tool, guiding individuals toward a balanced and nourishing lifestyle.

By introducing beginners to the principles of the Dietary Approaches to Stop Hypertension (DASH) diet, this cookbook equips them with the knowledge and skills necessary to make informed dietary choices. It demystifies the complexities of nutrition, offering clear and concise guidance on how to incorporate wholesome, nutrient-rich foods into everyday meals.

Moreover, the cookbook's emphasis on the right diet extends beyond mere calorie counting or restrictive eating habits. It promotes a holistic approach to nutrition, encouraging individuals to focus on the quality of their food rather than simply the quantity. By prioritizing whole, unprocessed ingredients, it fosters a profound sense of vitality and well-being that transcends the limitations of traditional dieting.

Furthermore, the Dash Diet Cookbook for beginners celebrates the joy of cooking and eating, inviting individuals to savor every moment of their culinary journey. It encourages experimentation and creativity in the kitchen, empowering beginners to discover new flavors and textures while staying true to the principles of the DASH diet.

As beginners navigate the pages of this cookbook and embark on their culinary adventure, they are not just learning to cook; they are embarking on a transformative journey toward better health and vitality. With each recipe mastered and every meal enjoyed, they are reclaiming control over their well-being and laying the foundation for a lifetime of health and happiness.

In essence, the Dash Diet Cookbook for beginners with the right diet is more than just a collection of recipes; it is a roadmap to a healthier, more vibrant life. So let us embrace this journey with open hearts and open minds, knowing that with each mindful bite, we are nourishing our bodies, minds, and spirits, one delicious meal at a time.